DEFEATING SCLERODERMA

30 Solutions to Overcome Scleroderma Symptoms for a Healthier and Happier Life

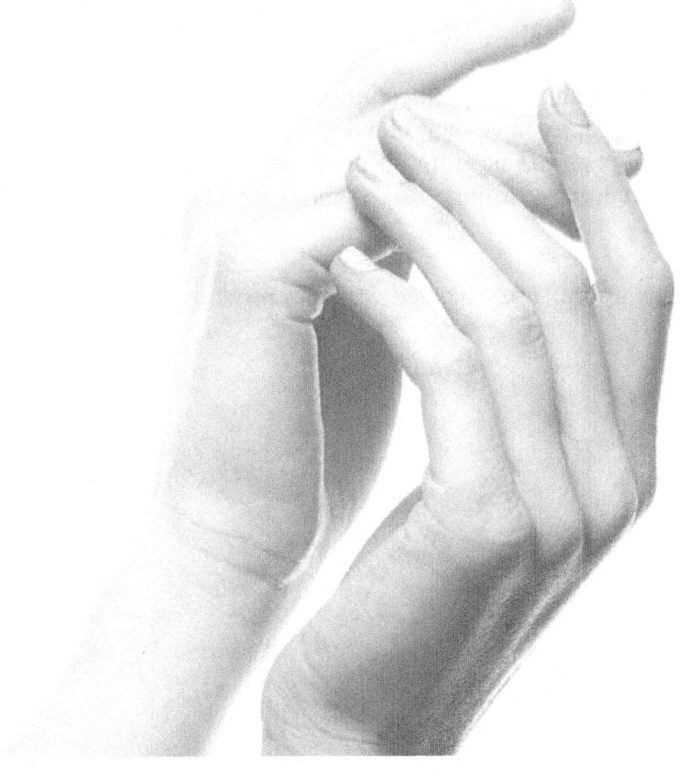

First Printing: 2020

Copyright © 2020 by Georgianne Micheals

The total or partial reproduction of this work is allowed as long as its origin is cited and it is for the personal use of the readers, without commercial purposes or lucrative spirit, without in these cases it is possible to alter, transform or generate a derivative work from of this work.

Authors and their publications mentioned in this work and bibliography have their copyright protection. All brand and product names used in this book are trademarks, registered trademarks, or trade names and belong to the respective owners.

The author is unassociated with any product or vendor in this book.

Contents

Intro Sclero-what?..11

1 What is scleroderma and why have I been diagnosed with it?...15
    The types of scleroderma 15
    What causes scleroderma...................................16
    Is there a cure?...17

2 Will there ever be a cure? 19
    Anti-inflammatory medications...........................19
    Immune suppressive therapy 20
    Treatment of vascular disease with drug therapy 20
    Anti-fibrotic drugs 21

3 What should I expect? 23
    Extreme tiredness...24
    Hardened and thickened skin 24
    Stiffened and painful joints.................................25
    Digestive issues..26

4 Morphea and scleroderma – are they the same thing?..29
    Signs and symptoms of morphea........................30
    Solutions for treating morphea..........................30

5 What does early detection mean? 33
How to find out if you have scleroderma...................33
What to do after a scleroderma diagnosis..................34

6 What does scleroderma mean for my skin?............37
Treatment of skin hardening and thickening..............38

7 What will happen to my joints and muscles? 41
Pain from joint stiffness..41
Arthritis..42
Joint contractures..42
Pain from stiffened tendons 43

8 Do massages help with joint and muscle pain? 45

9 Are there other methods for dealing with the pain? 47
Physical therapy..47
Acupuncture..48
Acupressure...48
Chiropractic care 48
More pain relief methods 49

10 Is my heart at risk? 51
How to prevent heart disease 52

11 Is kidney failure imminent?..53

How to keep your kidneys as healthy as possible ...54

12 How does scleroderma affect my lungs?...............57
Types of lung involvement..58
How to keep your lungs as healthy as possible.........59

13 How does Scleroderma affect my digestive system?..61

14 GERD – How is it related to scleroderma?.............63
Treatment for GERD..64

15 What is the best diet for scleroderma patients?..67
The best diet for scleroderma patients 69
Foods that should be avoided or reduced on the low FODMAP diet...70
Foods that are good to eat on the low FODMAP diet
....71
How to start the low FODMAP diet................................72

16 Bladder and bowel movements – What do I need to know? 73
Scleroderma and bowel movement...............................73
Solutions for dealing with scleroderma-induced bowel symptoms 75
How scleroderma affects the bladder..........................75

17 Should I exercise? If so, what types should I do? 77

Considerations that need to be made when exercising 78

The best exercises for scleroderma patients...............79

18 What other lifestyle changes should I make?........81

Developing a strong support system..........................81
Use sunscreen..82
Learn makeup application techniques........................82
Invest in daily living aids 82

19 Are there other diseases associated with scleroderma?..85

Lupus..85
Rheumatoid arthritis 86
Sjogren's syndrome..86
Fibromyalgia 87
Sexual dysfunction...87
Vasculitis..88
More diseases and medical conditions associated with scleroderma...89

20 Erythromelalgia vs Raynaud's phenomenon – What do I need to know? 91

What triggers erythromelalgia....................................92
Coexistence of erythromelalgia and Raynaud's phenomenon 92
How to treat erythromelalgia.....................................93

21 CREST – What do I need to know? 95
    Treatment for CREST..96

22 Migraines – another symptom? 99

23 How does scleroderma affect sexuality? 101
    Sexual dysfunction in men...................................101
    Sexual dysfunction in women..............................102
    General tips for improving sexual fulfillment for scleroderma patients..103

24 What does scleroderma mean for fertility? 105
    How scleroderma affects fertility in women 105
    How to decrease the risk factors associated with pregnancy..107

25 What is it like to be pregnant with scleroderma? 109
    How is a baby affected by scleroderma? 109
    Will scleroderma get worse during pregnancy?......110
    Can a woman with scleroderma have a natural birth? 111
    What happens after delivery?...............................111
    Can scleroderma patients breastfeed?..................112

26 Should I consider HSCT (Hematopoietic Stem Cell Transplant)? 113

27 How do I deal with the mental trauma? 115

28 How much will I be affected by fatigue? 117
   Natural remedies for fighting the chronic fatigue of scleroderma 118

29 Are there any natural remedies that help with the symptoms of scleroderma? 121
   Potassium para-amino benzoic acid 121
   Vitamin E 122
   Vitamin C 122
   Vitamin D 123
   Evening primrose oil 123
   More natural remedies 123

30 City or country living? Are some environments better suited for living with scleroderma? 125

Conclusion 127

Reference 129

Acknowledgments

Many thanks to my mentor Christopher John Payne at www.christopherjohnpayne.com, who has given me great advice on creating books and ebooks.

Also heartfelt thanks to my gorgeous partner who has been a tremendous source of encouragement and support.

About the Author

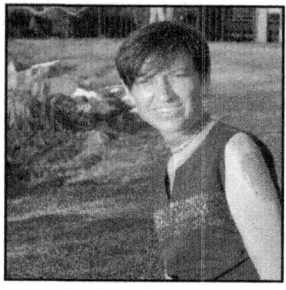

Georgianne Micheals

Georgianne's mission is to help both herself and other scleroderma sufferers by documenting her experiences with this disease as well as the solutions she has discovered to dealing with the pain.

When not documenting her journey with scleroderma, she creates sweet LGBT romances. As a bisexual woman, she has experienced the best of both worlds before she decided to settle down with her beloved female partner.

Intro

Sclero-what?

Scleroderma.

I had never heard the word before that fated day that my doctor diagnosed me with the disease. With the weight of so many syllables bearing down on me, I certainly felt panicked. I suppose anyone else would as well if being told that they were going to die sooner than later.

Let me back up a little and tell you what my life was like before that day.

I considered myself a normal woman who lived a somewhat boring life. I had watched my mother suffer from the autoimmune disease called systematic lupus erythematosus until she died when I was only 22 years old. As such, I am very health-conscious, determined to control my destiny and avoid the same path that my mother had suffered. That is why I exercised 3 days a week, ate fruits and veggies religiously, and downed the recommended daily intake of water. I knew my genetics played a part and there was still a likelihood that I would develop the same condition that my mother had. So focused on that one disease and actively trying to avoid sickness with impeccable life choices, this diagnosis completely blindsided me

I was diagnosed with scleroderma in early 2017. I subjected myself to a long list of tests yearly to ensure that I had dodged the bullet with systematic lupus erythematosus. Every year before that, I had come back with a clean bill of health. Skin biopsy, blood tests, urine tests, images taken with an MRI scan… You name it and I did it despite jokes from other family members that I was being paranoid.

Used to the routine, I was not even worried when I complained to my doctor about a simple condition that I had been suffering at that time. This had been tingling in my fingers along with intermittent feelings of numbness and the tips turning a slight blue color. I worked in IT as a server administrator. I was in air-conditioned rooms often and detested the cold for its effects on my body.

Even though scleroderma is derived from the Greek words that mean "hardness" and "skin", I have not even experienced that symptom. I looked at my life and turned my behavior over in my mind to see what had caused this but I could not trace this diagnosis to any specific behavioral pattern. I fell into a period of depression, I admit. I wondered why me and all the typical woes of being newly diagnosed with any health condition.

That is until I was reminded that I am me and I am not one to give up. I will certainly not give up my life to this disease. I will learn to manage it and to treat whatever symptoms that arise. That was my promise to myself. From that declaration rose my need to help other people who also suffer from scleroderma.

This book is a testament of my experiences with the disease thus far and an in-depth documentation of my search for answers in dealing with the symptoms. I have consulted with my licensed doctor and other medical professionals, read many books, scoured the internet, communicated with other scleroderma patients and more in my search.

There is a lot of misinformation and unfounded myths about scleroderma. I even came across a post about a man whose fingers turned rock-hard from this condition and fell off – all within 24 hours. I kid you not!

This made my initial search very stressful and daunting, and I am sure that many other persons experience the same emotions that I did. This book is a reliable resource that turns these myths and mistruths on their head and examines them to bring you the truth as well as reliable and effective solutions to deal with the symptoms of scleroderma.

Each chapter to follow commences with a question about a problem specific to scleroderma and solutions for dealing with that problem.

While this is indeed a terrible disease to deal with and there can be horrible pain involved, this disease does not define me, you or anyone else affected by scleroderma. There are effective solutions to deal with the symptoms and I will share them with you.

No two scleroderma patients suffer in quite the same way, which is why this disease is so hard to diagnose. Still, I endeavored to deliver solutions that work across the board whether you are newly diagnosed or a longtime sufferer, and for various levels of pain and suffering.

Before we jump in, I want to make it clear that the advice given in this book is not meant to supersede any of that given to you by your doctor. Only you and your doctor know your medical history and your particular needs. Remember to always consult with your doctor or other healthcare professionals before you make any change to your lifestyle.

Without further ado, let's get started.

1

What is scleroderma and why have I been diagnosed with it?

Scleroderma is an autoimmune, chronic, and rheumatic disease that manifests itself in the hardening of connective tissue within the body. That is a mouthful to say but essentially, this means that this is a disease in which the immune system overreacts and mistakenly attacks its own healthy cells because it thinks that they are foreign invaders such as bacteria and viruses.

This condition is chronic because it persists over a long period of time or reoccurs constantly. The rheumatic aspect of this disease is characterized by inflammation in the supporting structures of the body such as the joints, bones, and muscles.

The types of scleroderma

There are two main types of scleroderma. They are called localized and systemic scleroderma. Each of these categories is characterized by different conditions. Localized scleroderma affects only the skin. It is often considered the lesser evil of the two types of scleroderma as it does not affect major organs.

Systemic scleroderma, on the other hand, not only affects the skin but also hardens major organs and blood vessels. Persons with systemic scleroderma often have complications of the heart, lungs, kidneys, and gastrointestinal tract.

Scleroderma can manifest itself in many ways and as such, the severity of symptoms varies from person to person. While it might just be a mild annoyance to some patients, it might be life-threatening to others.

The early symptoms of scleroderma often occur in the fingers, as was with my case. Fingers may become sensitive to cold environments and change color to blue or white. This change of color may also be a response to emotional stress. This is a manifestation of Raynaud's phenomenon, a condition that we will discuss later on in this book.

You may also find that your fingers become puffy and stiff. These changes are a result of the narrowing of blood vessels due to excess collagen accumulation in the area. This causes the blood vessels to overreact in cold temperatures or situations where there is emotional distress.

What causes scleroderma

Doctors do not yet know what causes scleroderma to occur but there are risk factors that make a person more susceptible to being diagnosed with the disease. These risk factors include:

- Environmental triggers such as being exposed to certain medications, pollution, and viruses.

- Having another autoimmune disease such as lupus, rheumatoid arthritis, or Sjogren's syndrome. Almost 20% of scleroderma diagnoses arise after such problems have been indicated in patients.

- Genetics. Scleroderma runs in some families and may also arise within persons who have family members who display symptoms of other autoimmune diseases. Sex and ethnic background also play a role. Women, especially those of the African American community are more susceptible to developing scleroderma. 6 out of 7 scleroderma patients are women.

- Age. Persons between the ages of 20 and 50 years old are more likely to develop scleroderma but children and older adults are also susceptible to getting the condition.

Is there a cure?

The unfortunate truth is that the complications that can arise from this condition are many. They include dental problems, scarring of lung, kidney, and heart tissue, decreased sexual function, and digestive issues such as heartburn cramps, constipation and diarrhea.

The good news is that, compared to other diseases, the numbers of people who are diagnosed with scleroderma are low. Less than 100,000 people in the US are diagnosed with the autoimmune disease. Better news is that most of these cases do not involve the severe complications mentioned above.

This is the part where I get to how to solve this problem but, unfortunately there is no solution for getting over scleroderma. It is an incurable disease.

Do not let this truth bring you down though because while this may be an incurable disease it is still a manageable one. Think of it this way - many people suffer with chronic diseases such as heart disease, diabetes, and high blood pressure but they still manage to live happy and healthy because they manage their symptoms. The same can be done with scleroderma.

There are several treatment options for the many symptoms and this book discusses them. Some of these solutions need to be prescribed by a doctor but there are natural remedies that scleroderma patients can practice at home to lessen the severity of their symptoms. That in itself is a solution.

2

Will there ever be a cure?

While scleroderma is currently incurable just like most other autoimmune diseases, great strides have been made in scientific research as it pertains to finding a cure. Some of this research is focused on the workings of genes. While one of the risk factors for developing scleroderma is genetics, scientists have found that scleroderma is not a direct result of faulty genes. Instead, it is theorized that the disease is a result of flawed communication between genes and cells. This flawed communication is what causes the manifestation of scleroderma symptoms. This theory, and others, is what allows scientists and doctors to conduct further studies and clinical trials.

Even without a cure, scleroderma treatment options are wide and varied due to the varied nature of scleroderma symptoms. Such treatment options include:

Anti-inflammatory medications

Inflammation is one of the body's first defenses in the wake of injury or invasion by entities such as bacteria and viruses. Just as with any other autoimmune disease, this response can be over-sensitized in the case of scleroderma.

There are two types of inflammation as it pertains to scleroderma. The first type is more conventional and causes myositis, arthritis, and serositis. This is inflammation of the muscles, joints, and lining of organs like the heart and lungs respectively. This type of inflammation can be treated with traditional anti-inflammatory drugs like corticosteroids and NSAIDs (Nonsteroidal anti-inflammatory drugs).

The other type of inflammation does not respond to corticosteroids and NSAIDs, and is related to skin and tissue injury. Thus, more scientific study is needed to find effective treatment options.

Immune suppressive therapy

This is a type of drug therapy that lowers the body's natural immune response. This type of therapy is typically used to aid organ transplants so that the body does not attack the new organ as a foreign object. Autoimmune suppressive therapy is also a great treatment option for managing autoimmune disorders and conditions such as scleroderma. This type of treatment is only used in severe cases of scleroderma because there are potential risks in performing this therapy due to the lowered immunity of the body.

Treatment of vascular disease with drug therapy

Vascular disease, which is the abnormal function of blood vessels, is common and widespread with scleroderma patients. This disease mainly affects small and medium arteries and clinically manifests itself as Raynaud's phenomenon.

Blood supply is restricted when a person suffers from vascular disease and as such, tissues are not provided with adequate supplies of oxygen and nutrients. This can lead to serious complications such as the over activation of fibroblast (large, flat and elongated cells that help heal wounds) and an increased likelihood of developing tissue fibrosis (the development of excess tough connective tissue in an organ or in tissue).

Other complications such as spasms of blood vessels, blood clots, thickening of blood vessels, and even the blockage of blood vessels can also occur.

As a result, scleroderma patients who suffer from vascular disease often use vasodilator therapy to alleviate the symptoms. Vasodilator therapy is the use of drugs that dilate blood vessels to facilitate the effective flow of blood.

Anti-fibrotic drugs

Examples of such drugs include colchicine, dimethyl sulfoxide, D-penicillamine, and para-aminobenzoic acid (PABA). Their function is to reduce collagen production and to stabilize the already existing excessive tissue collagen.

3

What should I expect?

I was terrified when I received my scleroderma diagnosis. Considering that I had never heard of the condition before, I had no idea what I should expect and, of course, I imagined the worst-case scenarios right off the bat.

Of course, there are extreme cases of scleroderma where life expectancy goes down dramatically. However, that all depends on the severity of scleroderma symptoms and how quickly the disease progresses. As with any such life-changing news, the best thing to do for you and your family is to become educated.

Being educated allows you to become someone who is living with the disease rather than a victim of that illness. It allows you to be proactive rather than passive in your treatment and how you are influenced by this disease.

The first step in being proactive is knowing what to look for as the early signs and the symptoms of the progression of scleroderma. As with my case, the early symptoms were changes in the color of my fingers, which is known as Raynaud's phenomenon. I have discovered that there are ways to manage this such as giving up smoking because nicotine constricts blood vessels and worsens Raynaud's phenomenon. Wearing several layers of clothing also helps ward off the cold. Using compression gloves also helps.

Also, if you ever notice open sores on your fingers, be proactive and visit your doctor right away so that these do not become infected and make the problem worse.

Raynaud's phenomenon is not the only early sign, though. Below you will find a list of other common symptoms and solutions that you can employ to manage them.

Extreme tiredness

More than 9 in 10 scleroderma patients experience this symptom.

Solutions: Plan your day so that you can manage your fatigue and tiredness. Do the most strenuous task when you have the most energy. Take a rest when and if you need to and do not forget to list this time into your daily schedule.

Also, find other ways to relax and recharge. It is okay to take a break and rest.

Hardened and thickened skin

This is a typical symptom of scleroderma and often affects a person's self-image.

Solutions: Manage the appearance of your skin by using ointments or creams to keep your skin moisturized. Wearing gloves and avoiding the use of harsh soaps also help in retaining the moisture in the skin. Soaking your feet and hands in warm paraffin wax also helps soften hardened skin.

Stiffened and painful joints

This symptom can take away mobility and limit the quality of life.

Solutions: Employing simple exercises can help retain movements around joints and therefore, reduce stiffness and pain. This is commonly used in physiotherapy.

Here are 2 examples of such simple exercises:

- Neck rotations. Start in a sitting position with your back straight. Turn your head left then right looking over your shoulder. Repeat this several times and ensure that your head remains straight. Do not look up or down while you do this.

- Making a starfish with your fingers. Start by making a tight fist with your hand then stretch all your fingers out so that your fingers resemble a starfish. Hold this pose for 5 seconds before making a fist once more and repeating this exercise.

Be sure to ensure that your entire body benefits from exercising. To do this, you can employ gentle cardio exercises such as yoga, swimming, and walking.

Digestive issues

There is a wide range of digestive problems that can be experienced with scleroderma. The symptoms include difficulty swallowing, heartburn, indigestion, diarrhea, constipation, loss of appetite, weight loss, and dental problems.

Solutions: To combat difficulty swallowing ensure that your mouth does not get dry. Do this by staying hydrated and drinking lots of fluids throughout the day. Instead of drinking water, you can try drinking thicker drinks like milk, which are easier to swallow.

Consuming soft foods such as purees also helps you swallow easier. Consuming sour foods such as lemons makes your mouth produce more saliva, which makes it easier to swallow as well.

To deal with indigestion and heartburn, eat smaller meals more frequently rather than eating a huge meal one time. Ensure that you sit up straight while you eat. This allows gravity to aid your digestion. Also, avoid eating and drinking just before bedtime.

Diarrhea and constipation can be avoided by eating foods that are rich in fiber, drinking plenty of fluids, and speaking to your doctor if symptoms become worse.

Poor appetite and weight loss can be combated by eating small amounts often so that you can get the most nutritional value from the foods that you eat. Also, supplement your meals with vitamins and minerals.

To ward off dental problems such as dry mouth, sip water and chew gum often to activate saliva production. Practicing good oral hygiene helps prevent oral ulcers, which are common with scleroderma patients.

If you find the skin around your mouth is becoming tight, practice mouth exercises such as opening your mouth as wide as you can to keep the skin around your mouth as elastic as possible.

4

Morphea and scleroderma – are they the same thing?

Localized scleroderma and morphea are two terms that are often used interchangeably but they are not the same thing. Rather, morphea is just one type of localized scleroderma.

It is the most common type of localized scleroderma. It manifests itself in a few ways such as one or a few thickened patches of skin that are varying degrees of pigment in appearance. Most often, these patches of skin are smooth and shiny. These patches of skin can also have varying degrees of hardness. While morphea is most often painless, itching is a common complaint.

Sometimes, morphea occurs in straight lines. This is called linear morphea. Just like scleroderma, morphea usually displays symptoms between the ages of 20 and 50 years old, and most often in women. Most of the time, morphea symptoms first occur during pregnancy. The cause of morphea has yet to be discovered and it is not contagious. Morphea is most prevalent in Caucasian women.

Signs and symptoms of morphea

The first signs of morphea can include:

- A gradual change in the texture, shine and dryness of a particular area of skin.

- Purple or red oval patches on the skin.

- Patches that develop a white or lighter pigment in the center.

- Linear patches, particularly located on the legs and arms, in the case of linear morphea.

- Loss of hair in the affected area.

- Loss of sweat glands in the affected area.

Morphea can affect any part of the body. The good news is that morphea usually goes away on its own over time even though reoccurrences are common.

Solutions for treating morphea

Treatment options include medicated creams that contain high amounts of vitamin D to help soften the skin patches, and oral medications and light therapy in the case of widespread or severe morphea.

Ways in which you can naturally treat morphea at home include supplementing your diet with vitamin D and vitamin

E, and using lotions that contain shea butter or coconut oil to soften skin.

To soothe itchy skin, try out these options:

- Keep your skin moisturized with fragrance-free and additive-free lotions and creams.

- Take cool or lukewarm baths and showers. Limit these baths and showers to 10 minutes or less.

- Use fragrance-free and additive-free soaps to bathe and detergents to wash your clothes.

- Use cooling agents like menthol or calamine.

- Use a wet, cold cloth or ice pack on the itchy area.

- Take an oatmeal bath.

- Wear loose clothing to keep from irritating your skin.

- Stick to relatively cool environments. Extreme temperatures can cause flare-ups.

5

What does early detection mean?

Being diagnosed with scleroderma is indeed a scary affair but it is better to know sooner rather than later. This allows you an element of control instead of being a victim of the symptoms.

Early detection of scleroderma is not as frequent as it should be because this disease displays symptoms that are similar to several other medical ailments. The official diagnosis does, however, give the scleroderma patient and his or her family a sense of direction on how to move forward.

How to find out if you have scleroderma

If you or someone you know suspects that scleroderma is the underlying cause of symptoms, the first thing to do is speak to your doctor. Make a note of your symptoms, the frequency, and the times that they occur. Journaling is a great way to do this.

Since there is no single test to diagnose scleroderma, you need to prepare yourself to be thoroughly examined by your doctor. You need to also relay your family history so research that information if need be and keep it on hand.

Skin biopsy and blood tests will be performed but these tests alone are not enough to make a scleroderma diagnosis. Additional tests include but are not limited to:

- X-rays to determine if there are changes in bones, tissues, and organs.

- Echocardiogram to examine the structure and function of the heart.

- Electrocardiogram (EKG or ECG) to determine if there are changes in heart muscle tissue.

- CT chest scan to evaluate if there is lung involvement.

- Breathing tests to assess how efficiently the lungs are working.

- Motility studies to assess for gastrointestinal dysmotility, which is a condition whereby food contents do not move effectively through the digestive tract.

What to do after a scleroderma diagnosis

Early detection of scleroderma allows for the creation of a game plan. Typically, your doctor will direct you to a rheumatologist and dermatologist to conduct blood tests and other specialized tests to determine how severely the disease is currently affecting your organs.

Once you have received the results of these tests, you can then work on a treatment plan for your current symptoms. This plan involves recording the particular problem then specifying details for management.

A sample scleroderma plan looks like this:

Problem	**Management**
Sjogren's Syndrome (dry eyes and mouth)	Make water readily available for drinking. Administer eye drops at the prescribed time.
Difficult bowel movements and constipation	Visit dietician as recommended.
Esophageal reflux and heartburn	Use anti-acids after each meal. Sit upright during and after meals. Elevate head when sleeping.

6

What does scleroderma mean for my skin?

One of the most common visible symptoms of scleroderma is changes to the skin. One of the tests used to determine the extent to which the condition affects a patient's skin is called the modified Rodnan skin score (mRSS).

The physician carries out the test by doing palpitations of the skin to determine the degree of hardening that has occurred. This palpitation is done to 17 areas which include the hands, fingers, upper arms, forearms, chest, face, upper leg, lower leg, feet, and abdomen. Each area is scored between 0, which is normal and 3, which is severe.

After this test has been performed, the score is tallied with a maximum score of 51 possible.

The skin score is a very important indicator of how severe the scleroderma disease has progressed in a patient. Typically, the more a scleroderma patient's skin is affected, the more severe his or her particular case. This is not a definitive sign of the severity of a scleroderma case, though.

Skin gets tightened and thickened due to an overproduction of the protein called collagen. Skin is mainly affected by localized scleroderma and may manifest itself in the form of oval-shaped hardened patches that are often red or purple and begin to turn white towards the center. This is called generalized morphea.

Localized scleroderma may also manifest its self in the form of streaks or lines of hardened skin on the face, legs, and arms.

While it may be impossible to completely reverse the hardening of skin once the condition has developed, there are solutions for softening the skin. Your doctor may recommend medications such as steroids and methotrexate.

Treatment of skin hardening and thickening

However, here are a few at-home solutions that you can employ:

- Regularly apply moisturizer to your skin. Do this at least 3 times daily.

- Use moisturizers, creams, or oils that contain vitamin D and E to moisturize your skin. They help protect and nourish the skin as well as diminish scar tissue.

- Use evening primrose oil to moisturize the skin. This oil helps to reduce the appearance of roughness, wrinkles, dryness, thickness, and irritation of the skin.

- Use avocado oil to moisturize skin. This oil is highly moisturizing and is also an antioxidant, and anti-inflammatory.

- Use soy extract. Derived from soybeans, this agent is an antioxidant and helps to restore and soothe skin.

- Use gentle cleansers and exfoliators to cleanse your skin of dead cells.

- Do not take long hot showers as these dry out your skin and make them more susceptible to hardening.

- Do not use harsh soaps or other substances with harsh chemicals on your skin.

- Use sunscreen before you go outside.

- Use a humidifier especially during the winter months. This applies moisture to the air, which helps skin remain soft and supple.

- Exercise regularly to improve blood circulation. This increases the supply of oxygen and nutrients to the skin, which makes it less susceptible to hardening.

- Practice a healthy diet that eliminates junk food, processed food, refined carbohydrates, and alcohol. Ensure that you consume food with a lot of vitamins and antioxidants such as berries and vegetables.

The consumption of omega-3 fatty acids also helps. Omega-3 fatty acids are commonly obtained from eating seafood and fish. You can also purchase fish oils from your local store.

- Drink plenty of water to help your cells work more efficiently.

7

What will happen to my joints and muscles?

Pain is a common complaint with scleroderma patients. Not only can it be caused by ulcers and Raynaud's phenomenon, but it can also be caused by stiffness and swelling in joints and muscles. Pain in joints and muscles can come from different sources.

Pain from joint stiffness

Many scleroderma patients complain of hand stiffness that is particularly painful in the morning. The stiffness typically goes away as the person moves around and goes about their daily routine. This stiffness is caused by inflammation.

This inflammation can make the hand appear puffy and can also make it impossible to form a tight fist. This difficulty is known as the edematous phase of scleroderma. Many patients often confuse this with arthritis but it is actually due to leakage from small blood vessels.

This causes fluid to gather in the hands and fingers. This fluid retention can last anywhere from a few weeks to a few years but typically goes away on its own. Unfortunately, it is often replaced by thickening and tightening of the skin, which can cause the fingers to curl downward. The pain resulting from this can range from mild to severe.

This inflammation is not limited to the hands but can also be experienced in the wrists, elbows, shoulders, and knees. The best way to combat this is to stay in motion throughout the day.

Arthritis

Arthritis is a general term used to describe any disorder that affects joints. Osteoarthritis is the most common type of arthritis and typically affects persons as they get older.

Arthritis caused by scleroderma is different from other types of arthritis as it causes pain and stiffness of joints without inflammation, which is usually a precursor to other types of arthritis. As a result, the usual anti-inflammatory medications that are recommended for arthritis may not be effective with arthritis caused by scleroderma.

Joint contractures

Healthy joints have a wide range of motion that can be flexed inward, rotated, and extended outward. A joint contracture is one that does not have this wide range of motion and cannot be fully straightened. This condition is not only limited to the wrists but can also be experienced in the knees, ankles, feet, and even hips. Practicing daily exercises is one of the natural ways that you can keep a healthy range of motion in your joints.

Pain from stiffened tendons

Tendons of fibrous cords that attach muscles to bones. They allow the smooth motions of healthy functioning muscles via a tendon sheath that contains a small amount of fluid.

Unfortunately, persons who suffer from scleroderma also often suffer from tendonitis, which is inflammation of tendons. Normally, this is linked to acute injury such as over usage of tendons, particularly in sports.

In scleroderma patients, this inflammation is caused by the overreaction of the immune system. It most often occurs at the ankles, knees, and elbows. The pain from this can range from mild to severe. Treatment options include the application of heat, and taking anti-inflammatory medicines and NSAIDs.

8

Do massages help with joint and muscle pain?

Massage therapy is the practice of kneading and rubbing the body by applying gentle or strong pressure to muscles and joints in an effort to ease tension and pain using the hands. There are several types of massages and each type caters to a specific purpose and benefit. For example, Swedish massages are a gentle type of full body massage and is ideal for people who are sensitive to touch or have a lot of tension. On the other hand, deep tissue massage is not ideal for persons who are overly sensitive to pressure but is a good option if a person has chronic pain or a lot of muscle tension.

Deep tissue massage makes use of deep finger pressure and slow strokes to knead the deepest layer of muscles and connective tissue. Even though firm pressure is being apply, no pain or soreness should be experienced from the massage if it is being done correctly.

This is a full body massage and thus, the person being massaged needs to be dressed down to at least their underwear. Getting fully nude is common for this type of massage. This type of massage typically lasts between 1 hour and 90 minutes.

Defeating Scleroderma

As it relates to scleroderma, typically deep tissue massage is the usual recommendation. It is most often done with a gentle and tactile approach. This works best as it helps manage pain, increase blood circulation, and lessen the other symptoms of scleroderma.

The massage therapist is the individual who administers the massage. The skill of a massage therapist is an important factor in the results gained. If you decide on massage therapy as a way to deal with your pain, ensure that you discuss a massage program with your doctor and the massage therapist so that you can agree on tactile sensitivity and the areas that need the most work in advance.

When getting a massage, do not be afraid to voice how you feel in the session. This will help your massage therapist better assess your needs and apply the massage in the way that benefits you the most.

9

Are there other methods for dealing with the pain?

Pain from scleroderma does not only result from joints and muscles. It can come from other sources such as carpal tunnel syndrome and other nerve-related problems. Due to the many sources of pain with this disease, pain management is an important subject. There are many alternatives for dealing with pain.

Physical therapy

Also known as physiotherapy, physical therapy is the treatment of a disease, deformity, or injury via physical means such as heat treatment and exercise rather than the use of drugs or surgery. Massage therapy is a type of physical therapy. Patients of scleroderma should consult a physiotherapist in order to get the best results and to lower the risk of further injury while practicing the method of physical therapy chosen.

Physical therapy helps with stretching the skin, joints, and muscles in an effort to increase range of motion, improve posture, and prevent the loss of muscle strength and mass.

Pain management is encouraged by the release of endorphins, which are naturally produced hormones that are released in response to pain, exercise and emotional stimulation.

Acupuncture

Originally an ancient Chinese practice, acupuncture involves the insertion of fine needles through the skin at specific points to relieve pain or cure diseases. This is an alternative form of medicine and should never be practice by an unlicensed individual because malpractice can lead to injury or death. If you decide to use this form of alternative medicine to treat your pain, do thorough research to find a licensed individual in the field in your area.

Acupressure

This is similar to the practice of acupuncture but instead of the use of needles, the pressure is applied using fingertips. This is a safer practice that you can perform on yourself.

However, you may have difficulty applying the needed pressure with your own fingertips. Therefore, you may need to seek the help of others to perform this form of alternative medicine effectively. In addition to providing pain relief, this is a great practice for inducing relaxation.

Chiropractic care

This is a procedure that is performed by a doctor of chiropractic medicine (D.C.) and involves the manipulation or adjustment of the spinal column. Manipulation and adjustment can also be applied to joints in the legs, arms, and neck.

The practice of chiropractic care is founded on the belief that several diseases are triggered by pressure that is specifically located along the nerves of the spine.

More pain relief methods

Pain relief methods are wide and varied and it would be impossible to go in-depth into all of them in this book. Therefore, I am providing a list below that you can explore to find out which may work for you if you are someone who experiences pain with scleroderma symptoms.

Additional pain relief methods including:

- Self-hypnosis, which is a mind-body technique that forces a person into a self-induced state of deep relaxation.

- Deep breathing, which uses controlled breathing techniques to relax and dispel pain.

- Visualization, which involves using mental imagery to make pain more tolerable.

- Floatation therapy, which involves floating in a pool filled with Epsom salt in a space where light and sound are restricted.

- The Alexander technique, which helps to promote better posture and thus, lessen pain.

- Biofeedback therapy, which is a mind-body technique that uses auditory or visual feedback to gain control over involuntary body functions.

- Meditation, which is a self-induced state of deep consciousness.

10

Is my heart at risk?

While most scleroderma patients do not suffer from serious heart disease, it is still a possibility because scleroderma can cause scarring of the heart tissue. This scarring can lead to abnormal heartbeats, inflammation of the membranes surrounding the heart and congestive heart failure.

Scleroderma can also cause cardiovascular problems by raising blood pressure on the right side of the heart. This causes the heart to wear itself out and thus, can lead to heart failure.

Typically, heart disease occurs as a response to scleroderma in the latter stages of the disease. Scleroderma patients can monitor the disease's effect on their heart with regular examinations by the doctor and the performance of periodic tests such as electrocardiography and 3D echocardiography.

Most often in the cases where heart disease does develop in scleroderma patients, pre-existing conditions encourage this development. Such factors include family history and smoking.

How to prevent heart disease

It is imperative that you care for your heart to ensure that the risk of developing heart disease, whether or not you have scleroderma, is lowered. Ways in which this can be done include:

- Being smoke-free
- Managing your blood pressure
- Managing your cholesterol levels
- Managing your blood sugar levels
- Being consistently physically active
- Managing your weight
- Practicing a healthy diet

11

Is kidney failure imminent?

High blood pressure is a common symptom of scleroderma and thus, this places the kidneys at risk. This can occur in cases of systemic scleroderma and is called kidney or renal involvement. It can be mild or severe but typically early signs of kidney involvement include:

- High blood pressure

- Protein in the urine

- Abnormalities in blood tests

Without management, kidney failure is a possibility. Kidney failure is the situation that arises when the kidneys are no longer able to perform the important function of expelling waste products from the body.

This usually arises from scleroderma renal crisis. This is preceded by an abrupt rise in blood pressure and rapidly progresses to kidney damamge among the possible repercussions. Other symptoms include shortness of breath, chest pain, mental confusion, and visual interruptions. If this is not treated immediately, it can lead to death. Treatment comes in the form of renal dialysis.

While this is all very scary to contemplate, scleroderma does not mean an automatic sentence to kidney failure.

How to keep your kidneys as healthy as possible

It is not possible to control the effect that scleroderma has on your kidneys. However, there are things that you can do to keep this organ, which regulates pH, potassium, and salt levels as well as produce hormones that regulate blood pressure and the production of red blood cells, as healthy as possible. A healthily function kidney is less likely to be impacted by scleroderma compared to a damaged one.

A few of the ways you can keep your kidneys healthy include:

- Exercising regularly so that your heart performs at optimal and your blood pressure remains stabilized. Both of these conditions have an effect on how your kidneys perform. You do not have to do hardcore exercises. Simple cardio exercises like cycling, running, dancing, and walking work just fine.

- Monitor your blood pressure. There are blood pressure monitors that you can use right in the comfort of your home to do this. A healthy blood pressure reading is 120/80. If you consistently gain readings above 140/90, consult your doctor immediately.

- Ensure that your blood sugar levels remain low so that your kidneys are not forced to work harder to filter your blood. This reduces the risk of kidney damage.

- Drink a lot of fluids to help flush out toxins and salts from your kidneys.

- Manage your weight and eat a healthy diet. Being overweight or obese places a person at risk of developing several health conditions. One of these conditions is kidney disease.

- Do not smoke. Smoking slows down blood flow to your kidneys. This places them at greater risk for developing conditions such as cancer and crisis.

12

How does scleroderma affect my lungs?

Unfortunately, lung involvement occurs in around 80% of scleroderma patients. Even though the symptoms can be mild, lung involvement is the leading cause of death and disability with this disease.

The most common symptoms of lung involvement as it relates to scleroderma include shortness of breath and fatigue due to physical activity. Not everyone displays these symptoms especially because many scleroderma patients have limited physical activity due to the pain of the symptoms.

Scleroderma lung involvement can occur because of:

- Inflammation
- Damage to blood vessels leading to the lungs
- Scarring of lung tissue

Types of lung involvement

There are two main ways in which scleroderma affect lungs and the name of these conditions are called interstitial lung disease (ILD), which is also known as lung fibrosis and involves the thickening and stiffening of the lungs, and pulmonary artery hypertension (PAH), which involves increased pressure in the blood vessels in the lungs.

Lung fibrosis manifests itself in symptoms such as:

- Being out of breath while doing simple tasks
- A persistent dry cough
- Frequently feeling dizzy
- Difficulty taking deep breaths

If you have these symptoms, discuss them with your doctor immediately because the sooner that lung fibrosis is detected, the more likely it is that your body will respond to treatment.

Due to the increased blood pressure in the lungs as with PAH, less oxygen is delivered into the bloodstream. As such, not only are the lungs are affected but also all the other organs in the body. Symptoms of this condition include all of those mentioned for lung fibrosis and includes:

- Chest pains.
- Lips and skin turning a bluish color in the condition known as cyanosis.

- Heart palpitations.

- Racing pulse.

Again, these are symptoms that you need to discuss with your doctor so that the condition, if diagnosed, can be managed effectively with treatment that is personalized to your specific condition.

How to keep your lungs as healthy as possible

Simple measures that you can take to decrease the severity of lung involvement as it relates to scleroderma include:

- Not smoking.

- Avoiding passive smoke.

- Caring for your esophagus with measures such as not yelling excessively or swallowing pieces of food that are too large and not been chewed properly.

- Being consistently physically active.

13

How does Scleroderma affect my digestive system?

Apart from the skin, the digestive system is the most commonly affected organ in patients suffering from scleroderma. Over 90% of scleroderma patients report symptoms that are related to the digestive system. Typical symptoms include abdominal pain, nausea, heartburn, diarrhea, constipation, difficulty swallowing (dysphagia), and lack of control over urination or defecation (incontinence). These symptoms can clearly affect a person's quality of life and their day-to-day activities.

These issues are primarily caused by a decreased blood supply to the nerves that feed the digestive system. This results in weakening of the muscles and therefore, slows down and disorganizes the motions of the gut. Typically, these symptoms start to perpetrate themselves in the esophagus and work their way down to the stomach and intestines.

The esophagus transports food from the mouth to the stomach with coordinated contractions of its muscular lining. These contractions are an automatic body function and typically, people are not aware that the body performs it except when pain is caused by swallowing something too large, eating too quickly or swallowing food or drinks that are extremely hot or cold. During these circumstances, of course, people feel the movement of food or drink down the esophagus and into the stomach. Of course, during these conditions, sensations of discomfort are experienced.

Most scleroderma patients who report problems with the digestive system are commonly referring to problems that affect the esophagus. The most common problem is heartburn.

Heartburn, is a symptom of GERD (gastroesophageal reflux disease). This condition produces a burning sensation in the chest due to acid regurgitation from the stomach into the esophagus. We will go more in-depth in to the topic of GERD in the next chapter.

Other symptoms that persist due to scleroderma's effect on the digestive system include reoccurring chest pain, mouth ulcers, an acidic taste in the mouth, and a persistent hoarse voice.

The easiest way to deal with problems with the esophagus is to eat pureed foods, drink smoothies and drink plenty of fluids as they are easier to swallow. Do not eat spicy, salty, or acidic food as they can trigger acid regurgitation into the esophagus.

14

GERD – How is it related to scleroderma?

GERD stands for gastroesophageal reflux disease. The main symptom of GERD is heartburn but other symptoms can be experienced as well. They include nausea, vomiting, respiratory issues, difficulty swallowing, and bad breath.

If left untreated, GERD can worsen into conditions such as:

- Esophageal stricture, which is the narrowing of the esophagus.

- Esophagitis, which is inflammation of the esophagus.

- Barrett's esophagus, which is the transformation of cells lining the esophagus into cells similar line in the intestines. This is a serious condition that can develop into cancer.

- Respiratory issues caused by the breathing in of stomach acid into the lungs.

GERD is a common condition even without the underlying issue of scleroderma. However, a scleroderma diagnosis can trigger the development of this condition.

Treatment for GERD

There are medications that can be used to treat GERD and surgery can be performed in extreme cases to prevent the reflux of acid into the esophagus.

Milder treatments for this condition stems around controlling the amount of acid that is produced in your stomach as well as conditions that might cause regurgitation of acid into the esophagus.

Ways in which you can do this include:

- Wearing loose clothing around your abdomen so that acid is not pushed from the stomach and up into the esophagus.

- Staying upright for at least 3 hours after eating meals.

- Sleeping at an angle with your head elevated.

- Not overeating.

- Eating at least 3 hours before bedtime.

- Managing your weight so that you are not neither overweight nor underweight.

- Avoiding alcoholic drinks.

- Avoiding spicy and fatty foods, chocolate, peppermint, caffeine-containing products, foods that contain tomato ingredients, and a peppermint.

- Using antacids.

- Not smoking and avoiding second-hand smoke.

15

What is the best diet for scleroderma patients?

Diet, meaning the food that we eat, is the single most influential factor that affects our health whether it be in a good or bad way. The impact of diet is multiplied when a person has a potentially life-threatening illness like scleroderma. Difficult swallowing and loss of appetite can make it difficult for a scleroderma patient to get the proper nutrition he or she needs to not only be generally well but to also fight this disease.

If you have difficulty swallowing, try:

- Pureeing fruits and vegetables to eat.

- Make smoothies using fruits, vegetables, seeds, nuts and nut butters, protein powders and more to get a wide variety of nutrients.

- And eat moist and soft protein sauces like scrambled eggs, ground meats and creamy casseroles.

Loss of appetite can lead to malnutrition. Signs of malnutrition include:

- Rapid weight loss within a 3-month period.

- The rapid decline of muscle mass.

- Weakness.

- Weakened immunity (getting sick with viruses like the common cold easily and frequently).

- Slow-healing wounds.

- Excessive hair loss.

- Brittle nails.

The first thing to do if you suffer from a low appetite is to realize that this is not your fault. Next, realize that there are ways to stimulate your desire to eat. Such ways include:

- Eating in situations that distract you from the act of eating like in social situations.

- Eating your favorite foods to whet your appetite.

- Avoiding eating foods that have strong odors to prevent nausea.

- Eating smaller meals more frequently.

- Increasing fiber intake and limit caffeine intake to prevent constipation.

- Trying natural remedies to stimulate appetite. Options include cloves, green tea, garlic, cayenne pepper, fennel, cardamom, and ginseng.

The best diet for scleroderma patients

There is no specific diet that works for scleroderma because the symptoms of the disease vary from patient to patient. However, there are a few guidelines that can be followed to minimize the most severe and frequent symptoms, as well as stabilize collagen production. These guidelines include:

- Eating small meals every 3 to 4 hours instead of 3 huge meals.

- Eat fresh, whole foods like fruits and vegetables instead of processed foods.

- Eliminate foods with added sugars from your diet. You can still eat foods that have sugars naturally like milk, yogurt, and fruit.

- Eat foods that are rich in antioxidants like berries.

- Eat anti-inflammatory foods like basil, curry powder, ginger, oregano, cinnamon, turmeric, and rosemary.

- Add a multi-vitamin to your diet as a supplement.

The low FODMAP diet is one that falls within the parameters of the dietary requirements for most scleroderma patients. FODMAP stands for **F**ermentable, **O**ligosaccharides like fructans, **D**isaccharides like lactose, **M**onosaccharides **A**nd **P**olyols like sugar alcohols such as sorbitol. Oligo-, di-, mono-saccharides and polyols are groups of carbohydrates that are known to aggravate digestive problems like stomach pain, bloating and gas.

This diet is great for scleroderma suffers because it decreases flare-ups of the digestive issues by restricting the consumption of high FODMAP foods. It is a common recommendation for people who suffer from irritable bowel syndrome (IBS) as well.

Foods that should be avoided or reduced on the low FODMAP diet

- Vegetables and legumes like onion, red kidney beans, taro, split peas, celery, cassava, asparagus, artichoke, black-eyed peas, cauliflower, mushrooms, lima beans, fermented cabbage, beetroot and falafel.

- Fruits that have a high fructose value like avocados, dates, grapefruits, watermelon, peaches, mango, plums, currants, figs, mango, guava, cherries, and pears.

- Cereals, pasta, nuts, breads, cookies, and biscuits that contain wheat.

- Highly processed poultry, meat and meat substitutes like sausages.

- Dairy foods like buttermilk, cream cheese, ice-cream, sour cream, milk, and custard.

- Sweeteners, dips, spreads, and condiments like agave, fruit bars, honey, molasses, hummus, tahini, jam, and gravy that contains onion.

- Protein powders.

- Drinks like beer, coconut water, rum, fruit juices, teas, and wine.

Foods that are good to eat on the low FODMAP diet

- Vegetables and legumes like okra, parsnip, olives, pumpkin, seaweed, chickpeas, carrots, callaloo, black beans, chives, cucumbers, kale, green peppers, zucchini, squash, spinach, and yam.

- Fruits like tamarind, strawberry, dragon fruit, ackee, green bananas, kiwi, honeydew, lemon, mandarin, and passion fruit.

- Minimally processed poultry, meat and meat substitutes like pork, lamb, turkey, chicken, and beef.

- Fish and seafood like tuna, salmon, cod, crab, shrimp, and lobster.

- Wheat-free and gluten-free cereals, pasta, nuts, breads, cookies, and biscuits.

- Sweeteners, dips, spreads, and condiments like almond butter, chocolate, mustard, soy sauce, vinegars, stevia, and marmalade.

- Dairy foods like eggs, tempeh, margarine, butter, brie, and feta cheese.

How to start the low FODMAP diet

Practicing the low FODMAP diet follows a specific regimen. It goes like this:

Stage 1: It is called Restriction and involves absolute avoidance of all high FODMAP foods.

Stage 2: This stage is about the systematic Reintroduction of high FODMAP foods to determine the type of high FODMAP food you are sensitive to and the amount of high FODMAPS you can tolerate. This tolerance is called your threshold level.

Stage 3: This stage is called the modified low-FODMAP diet because it is about personalizing your diet based on the tolerances identified in stage 2.

16

Bladder and bowel movements – What do I need to know?

The bowels are composed of the small intestine, large intestine, colon and rectum. As part of the digestive system, the function of the bowels is to help the body absorb nutrients from food and fluids ingested as well as expel any waste produced in the digestive process.

Scleroderma symptoms can affect the bowels as well as the bladder with symptoms such as constipation, diarrhea, fecal incontinence, and urinary incontinence. We will take a look at how scleroderma affects the bowel and bladder individually and any possible solutions for dealing with these problems below.

Scleroderma and bowel movement

A normally functioning small intestine allows for the most absorption of nutrition from the food and liquids that are ingested. After this extraction is done, the waste products are propelled in to the large intestine to be excreted as fecal matter through the rectum.

Scleroderma affects this normal function by causing deterioration of the muscles in the organs. This leads to the stagnation of food in both intestines. The stagnation causes the production of bacteria in a condition known as small intestinal bacterial overgrowth (SIBO). This bacteria uses up the nutrients provided by the food ingested and thus, leads to nutritional deficiencies, weight loss, and malnutrition in the patient. This can induce symptoms such as vomiting, nausea, bloating, and abdominal pain.

Scleroderma can also incite the symptom known as pseudo obstruction. This is a condition whereby the bowels are not physically blocked but exhibit symptoms as if this is the case because the muscles simply stop functioning or function minimally. This can lead to scleroderma patients experiencing vomiting, inability to pass gas, abdominal pain and abdominal distension. Abdominal distension is the enlargement of the abdomen.

The large intestine is also affected by the weakening of muscles, which causes impaired mobility of waste products. The stagnation can lead to constipation, which is a condition whereby a person has less than 3 bowel movements per week.

A scleroderma patient may also be affected by the symptoms of diarrhea from impacted stool in the colon. This arises due to inflammation along the lining of the colon. Diarrhea is loose and watery stool.

Bowel incontinence, which is the condition whereby a person accidentally soils themselves before being able to make it to the bathroom, occurs in over 30% of all scleroderma patients. This occurs due to the weakening of the rectal muscles.

Solutions for dealing with scleroderma-induced bowel symptoms

- The solutions outlined for dealing with GERD also apply for bowel symptoms of scleroderma.

- Using stool softeners and practicing a liquid diet can help with constipation.

- Practicing a high fiber diet may help with constipation as well.

- Prescribed antibiotics can help with bacterial infections.

- Antibiotics can also be used to treat diarrhea as well as drinking a lot of fluids and eating items such as bananas, applesauce, and toast.

- A patient may be able to get relief from bowel incontinence by practicing biofeedback therapy.

How scleroderma affects the bladder

Scleroderma can weaken the muscles of the pelvic floor, which is where the bladder sits. This can lead to symptoms such as frequent urination and urinary incontinence, which is the inability to hold it in before making it to the bathroom.

Urinary incontinence can also be caused by constipation, which places extra pressure on the bladder.

One of the best solutions for fighting these two symptoms includes gaining better control of the muscles that surround the bladder. Pelvic floor muscle strengthening exercises can be practiced. One of the best-known exercises is called Kegels exercises, which simply involves the tightening and relaxing of the Kegel muscles for a few second intervals.

Also, drinking adequate amounts of liquids can help to decrease urine concentration, which can cause bladder irritation and infection. Reduce the amount of caffeinated and carbonated drinks that you consume.

If you have urinary incontinence, consider aids such as pads or adult diapers to avoid the embarrassment of wetting your underwear.

If bladder problems persist, be sure to talk to your doctor about investigating further solutions. Your doctor can also prescribe antibiotics in the case of bladder infections.

17

Should I exercise? If so, what types should I do?

Exercise can be a vital tool for scleroderma symptoms management but only after it has been cleared with your doctor. If you have the following conditions, do not partake in any exercise routine until you have discussed it with your doctor:

- Taking any medication that requires rest or that affects balance.

- Severe joint or muscle pain.

- Experiencing a flare period.

- Experiencing extreme or debilitating fatigue.

- Experiencing high blood pressure before exercise begins.

- Experiencing new or unexplained symptoms.

- Have difficulty breathing.

- Experiencing headaches.
- Have unexplained weight changes.

Considerations that need to be made when exercising

After you have made all due considerations and have been cleared to exercise by your doctor, here are a few tips to get the most out of your workout sessions:

- Be mindful of your range of motion to prevent joint pain and deformities.
- Be mindful when handling weights to prevent joint pain and deformities.
- Allow enough rest between sets of exercise.
- Allow enough rest between weekly workout sessions to ensure adequate recovery time.
- Be mindful of the amount of energy that you have daily to ensure that you can complete other tasks throughout the day.
- Be mindful of hygiene and cleanliness to ensure that no infections arise.
- Keep a detailed record of any symptoms experienced during exercise.

- Keep your workouts individualized to get the most benefit.

The best exercises for scleroderma patients

Aerobic exercises are the best type of exercise approved for scleroderma patients. They are more commonly known as cardio exercises because they increase breathing and heart rate for the duration of the activities. Cardio exercises help keep the lungs, heart, and circulatory systems healthy as well as get you moving.

They are not too tasking on the body and can be sustained for longer periods of time, which is a sharp contrast to anaerobic exercises such as sprinting and weightlifting, which involve quick bursts of energy.

Aerobic exercises can also be combined with resistance exercises to improve muscle strength and endurance. Resistance exercises are performed by moving your limbs against some sort of resistance like your own body weight, dumbbells or bands. Pushups, lunges and step-ups are examples of resistance exercises. Be sure to not overdo if you practice resistance exercises.

Examples of easy aerobic exercises that can be done at home or without the assistance of a personal trainer include:

- Jump rope
- Running

- Walking
- Jogging

Examples of aerobic gym exercises include:

- Swimming
- Using a stationary bike
- Using the treadmill

Aerobics class workouts are also available if you feel the need to have a supportive and encouraging environment while exercising. Aerobics class workout types include cardio kickboxing, indoor cycling classes, and Zumba.

18

What other lifestyle changes should I make?

Management of scleroderma symptoms can only be done on an individualized basis. However, there are general lifestyle changes that you can implement no matter what your symptoms are. Such measures include:

Developing a strong support system

The impact of suffering from scleroderma is not only limited to physical symptoms but mental and emotional symptoms as well. Having a strong support system such as supportive friends, family, and healthcare providers, is essential to remaining positive and developing the best outlook when dealing with this disease.

Enlisting the help of a therapist is also a great idea to help you navigate the psychological and emotional changes that accompany a diagnosis of such a disease.

There are also support groups, both in-person and online, that can aid. Spending time with others who understand the severity of the consequences of being diagnosed with scleroderma can help ease the emotional toll.

Use sunscreen

Many people with scleroderma have a sensitivity to sunlight. Using a gentle sunscreen, particularly one that lists PABA as one of the ingredients, will help you when you want to enjoy time in the sun.

Learn makeup application techniques

The physical signs and symptoms such as skin irritation and discoloration can make scleroderma patients feel very self-conscious. Learning tips and tricks to camouflage these problem areas with makeup can lessen this self-consciousness and allowing scleroderma patients to feel more comfortable when venturing outside of the home or comfort zones.

Invest in daily living aids

Consider mobility aids if scleroderma affects your ability to get around. Walking trolleys are a good investment if mobility is an issue for you.

Another issue may be comfort when sitting. Therefore, investment in footrests and reclining chairs should also be a consideration.

If skin becomes too tight or sore skin in the hands, gripping may become an issue. There are grip helpers such as pen grippers, foam tubing, food preparation aids, and other tools that help with gripping.

19

Are there other diseases associated with scleroderma?

Because of the possible widespread nature of scleroderma, it is associated with many other diseases and health conditions. Below you will find the name, a brief description of some of these, and any possible solutions for preventing or minimizing the symptoms of each.

Lupus

More precisely known as systemic lupus erythematosus (SLE), lupus is an autoimmune condition that is characterized by inflammation that damages muscles, joints, kidneys, and other organs. Around 1 in 5 people who suffer from scleroderma also have a crossover to this condition.

Even though anyone can develop lupus, it is most prevalent in women in their childbearing years. Triggers for the development of the condition range from puberty, menopause, or following childbirth or some other trauma.

There is no cure for lupus as with many autoimmune diseases but your doctor can place you on a good treatment plan that includes anti-inflammatory drugs, immune suppressants, and steroids to fight the most severe symptoms like fatigue, hair loss, Raynaud's phenomenon, and butterfly rash over the cheeks.

Rheumatoid arthritis

This is a chronic autoimmune condition that is characterized by inflammation that most commonly affects joints. The damage is typically not limited to joints and can include blood vessels, heart, lungs, eyes, and skin. Common warning signs of the development of this condition include fatigue, joint stiffness, joint pain, joint swelling, weight loss, and fever.

Treatment options include the use of NSAIDs, steroids, and disease-modifying anti-rheumatic drugs (DMARDs).

Sjogren's syndrome

Named after Henrik Sjogren, a Swedish ophthalmologist, this is an autoimmune immune disorder in which the immune system attacks glands that produce fluids in the body. It commonly occurs together with scleroderma as well as with lupus and rheumatoid arthritis. The condition typically occurs more commonly in women than in men and is usually diagnosed between the ages of 40 and 60 years.

Because this syndrome primarily affects tear glands and salivary glands, dry eye and mouth are common symptoms of this disease. Fatigue is also a common symptom. In severe cases of this condition, the kidneys, heart, brain, and lungs can also be affected.

Eye drops and anti-inflammatory medication are typical treatment options. Dietary changes such as moistening food with added dressings or sauce, avoiding spicy, acidic and salty food, and frequently sipping water can also help.

Fibromyalgia

This is also known as fibromyalgia syndrome. It is a chronic condition in which the primary symptom is pain that occurs all over the body. Even though the actual cause of fibromyalgia is not yet known, this condition often results after suffering some type of trauma such as a fall, viral infection, operation, or childbirth.

Other symptoms include stiffness all over the body, fatigue, tenderness to touch, sexual dysfunction, mood disturbances, anxiety, inability to concentrate, dizziness, headaches, and hypersensitivity to temperature changes. Diagnosis for this condition is difficult and as such, you need to immediately discuss it with your doctor if you experience these symptoms.

Sexual dysfunction

Many men with systemic scleroderma experience erectile dysfunction. This is a result of damage to blood vessels supplying the groin. This may result in the development of the condition known as Peyronie's disease. This is a non-cancerous condition that arises due to fibrous scar tissue developing on the penis. It causes curved and painful erections.

Women with scleroderma can also experience sexual dysfunction. This is particularly in the case where the woman also has Sjogren's syndrome. The syndrome causes dysfunction in the mucus-producing membranes of the vagina, resulting in less lubrication when the woman is aroused. Less lubrication equates to possible pain and discomfort during sexual intercourse.

It is best that both men and women discuss these conditions with their doctors to determine the best course of action moving forward.

Vasculitis

This is a condition whereby blood vessels become inflamed because they are being attacked by the immune system. This results in changes in blood vessels such as weakening, narrowing, and scarring. This damage restricts blood flow and results in tissue and organ damage.

This condition can be acute (short term) or chronic (long lasting). The exact cause of this condition is not yet known but it is often triggered by chronic infections like hepatitis C and hepatitis B.

Symptoms include headache, fever, fatigue, weight loss, general aches and pains, night sweats, and rashes. Nerve problems such as weakness and numbness can also occur. Again, this is something that needs to be discussed with your doctor so early diagnosis can be done if you are a sufferer of vasculitis. Then, a treatment plan can be developed to include the appropriate medications and therapies.

More diseases and medical conditions associated with scleroderma

As mentioned before, because of the widespread nature of the scleroderma on the body, the associated diseases and medical conditions are also varied. Those listed above are just a few, and others include pulmonary embolism. The best solution for preventing or treating any of these diseases is being constantly monitored by your healthcare provider so that diagnosis can be done as soon as possible should any of these conditions arise. Only then can treatment be implemented.

20

Erythromelalgia vs Raynaud's phenomenon – What do I need to know?

Erythromelalgia occurs rarely and is characterized by symptoms such as redness and pain in the feet mainly. This pain and redness can also be experienced in the legs, hands, arms, face, and ears. Pain can range on the scale from mild to burning. Therefore, simple activities like standing, walking, exercise, sleeping, and even social interaction can become difficult.

Clearly, this condition can have a severe impact on a person's quality of life. Other symptoms of this condition include:

- Swelling of the affected part of the body.

- Purple discoloration after the pain and redness has disbursed.

- Sweating in the affected area.

What triggers erythromelalgia

This condition can be triggered by an increase in body temperature. Body temperature can be increased for any variety of reasons such as after exercising, eating spicy food, drinking alcohol, being dehydrated, entering a warm room, or even wearing clothing such as socks or gloves.

Erythromelalgia is often a result of another underlying condition such as the blood disorder known as polycythemia, nerve damage, and other autoimmune diseases such as lupus or rheumatoid arthritis. Sometimes it is caused by a genetic problem.

Coexistence of erythromelalgia and Raynaud's phenomenon

Since these two conditions seem like they are opposite ends on a spectrum (one being triggered by heat and the other being triggered by exposure to cold temperature), erythromelalgia and Raynaud's phenomenon certainly do not seem like two conditions that would affect one person. However, there have been reports that these two conditions can coexist in the same scleroderma patient. The great news is that since erythromelalgia is such a rare condition, this coexistence hardly ever happens.

How to treat erythromelalgia

There are, of course, medications to treat this condition such as sprays, patches, gels, and creams. These topical medications make the skin less reactive to the heat receptors.

There are also oral medications and treatments options such as:

- Aspirin.

- Prescription-only painkillers.

- Blood pressure drugs to increase blood flow or decrease blood flow depending on the cause of this condition.

- Dietary supplements like magnesium, which dilates blood vessels.

There are other ways you can ease the symptoms of erythromelalgia at home and such methods include elevating the affected part of the body to decrease blood flow and using cool gel, cool packs, cool water, a fan or cool surface to cool down. Staying in air-conditioned spaces as much as possible also helps.

Be mindful that you should not use anything that is too cold or ice to cool down. Neither should you soak your hands or feet in cold water for too long of a period.

The first danger is that such an extreme drop in temperature can trigger a flare-up of erythromelalgia symptoms when the area warms up again.

Secondly, this exposure can lead to hypothermia, which is a dangerous condition where the body temperature drops below 35 degrees C. The normal temperature of a healthily functioning body is 37 degrees C. Hypothermia can lead to skin damage and, in extreme cases, the need for amputation.

21

CREST – What do I need to know?

CREST is a type of scleroderma known as limited scleroderma. Limited scleroderma is a sub form of systemic scleroderma. This type of scleroderma is diagnosed if a person has at least two of the following symptoms are listed below:

- **C**alcinosis, which is painful lumps of calcium in the skin.

- **R**aynaud's phenomenon.

- **E**sophageal dysfunction, which involves difficult swallowing and/or acid reflux. This occurs as a result of scarring in the esophagus.

- **S**clerodactyly, which is tightening and thickening of the skin on the fingers or toes. This condition can make it difficult to bend your fingers.

- **T**elangiectasias, which is red spots on the hands, forearms, palms, face, and lips, caused by blood vessel involvement.

Limited scleroderma is a milder form of the disease and every sufferer has a different pattern of symptoms. Typically, this type of scleroderma affects Caucasians.

While this is another form of scleroderma is milder, complication can arise. Examples include:

- Gastrointestinal issues. This is caused by scarring of the esophagus, which leads to difficulty swallowing and chronic heartburn. If this problem extends to the intestines it can cause diarrhea, constipation, bloating, weight loss, and malnutrition.

- Ulcers on the toes and fingers. This can arise due to the narrowing or abnormal function of blood vessels due to severe Raynaud's phenomenon. In extreme cases, this can lead to gangrene on fingers and toes, which will require amputation.

- Dry eyes and mouth.

Just like other types of systemic scleroderma, limited scleroderma can also lead to lung damage, kidney failure, heart problems, and dental issues.

Treatment for CREST

The focus with treating CREST, just like with other any type of scleroderma, is about relieving the symptoms and preventing complications. Therefore, treatment options include:

- Medications such as antacids for heartburn, topical antibiotics for ulcers, and blood pressure-lowering drugs.

- Therapy such as physical therapy to help prevent loss of mobility in fingers and occupational therapy such as special teeth brushing practices to care for teeth.

- Surgery such as the removal of calcium deposits and laser surgery to reduce the appearance of red spots and lines.

22

Migraines – another symptom?

Headaches and migraine are both symptoms of scleroderma by virtue of the fact that patients often suffer from elevated blood pressure among other symptoms. Migraines and headaches may also be a result of inflammation around the brain. Such inflammation is called cerebritis. This is a common symptom of lupus sufferers but can also affect scleroderma sufferers.

Migraines are a type of headache that include symptoms such as reoccurring throbbing on one side of the head. This pain can extend to other parts of the head and face. This problem is often accompanied by disturbed vision and nausea. Migraines can be triggered by other conditions such as insufficiently fluid intake, poor posture, changes in diet, medication side effects, hormonal changes, emotional triggers like stress, and environmental changes.

Migraines are complicated to deal with and as such, there is no one single sure, especially in the case of underlying issues like scleroderma. Still, there are measures that can be implemented to reduce the frequency of their occurrence. Such measures include:

- Considering the practice of a gluten-free diet. Gluten is a protein that is found in grains like barley, rye, or wheat. The link between gluten and migraines is not well understood but it is certainly there.

- Drinking plenty of water.

- Getting enough sleep. A well-rest brain is better able to combat changes in blood pressure.

- Reducing stress triggers in your environment.

- Exercising regularly.

- Speaking to your doctor about medications that may be triggering migraines so that alternatives can be sought.

- Consuming omega-3 fatty acids by eating seafood and fish.

- Consume anti-inflammatory herbs like turmeric and ginger.

23

How does scleroderma affect sexuality?

Scleroderma can cause sexual impairment in both men and women. This is heartbreaking because sexual function is an important part of healthy living and is a major contributor to a healthy romantic relationship.

Just as with anything that relates to the topic of sex, it is often a topic that is not openly discussed and so, many people are not aware of the problems and options for treating them. This chapter aims at providing a frank outline of the details and solutions that can be employed.

Sexual dysfunction in men

Erectile dysfunction is common in males who suffer from scleroderma. This is typically a result of local tissue fibrosis of the corpus cavernosum. The corpus cavernosum is a mass of erectile tissue that constructs the bulk of the penis and the clitoris. The function of this mass of tissue is to facilitate erections of the penis in men.

Erectile dysfunction can also be caused by abnormal microvascular function, which is associated with improper blood flow to the penile region.

Both conditions can cause pain and dry membranes in the groin in addition to the emotional and mental toll of sexual dysfunction.

Men who experience sexual dysfunction need to speak to their doctor frankly and openly so that their particular condition can be evaluated and proper treatment can be dispensed.

Sexual dysfunction in women

Sexual dysfunction in women can manifest itself in several ways. The first way is that many women who suffer from scleroderma often feel too tired to partake in sexual activities. Another way in which this can manifest itself is less lubrication of the vagina during arousal. This can make sex discomforting and even painful. Also, certain sexual position can cause discomfort and induce symptoms like acid reflux such as if a woman is lying flat on her back and has the weight of another body on top of her.

Ways in which women can combat sexual dysfunction include:

- Pacing themselves and resting up in anticipation of sexual activity.
- Using vaginal lubricants.

- Exploring new sexual positions that are more comfortable and do not trigger scleroderma symptoms.

General tips for improving sexual fulfillment for scleroderma patients

Sexual impairment can be disheartening for anyone but here are a few personalized tips for scleroderma patients to improve their sex life:

- Consult with your doctor to find out if the medications that you are using for treatment may be negatively impacting your sexual performance.

- If you feel loss of interest in sex or have problems becoming aroused due to depression and other mental problems, consult with your doctor to begin treatment for these.

- Avoid drinking alcohol before sexual activities.

- Avoid having a huge meal before sexual activities.

- Avoid sexual activities if you will feel very tired.

- Ensure that the atmosphere is calming and relaxing.

- Do not be afraid to explore more sexual positions that make both you and your partner feel more comfortable.

24

What does scleroderma mean for fertility?

Men and women experience different conditions as it relates to fertility and scleroderma. While men may experience erectile dysfunction and the performance issues as it relates to sexual activity, this in no way relates to a man's ability to conceive a baby as long as his sperm count and sperm quality are normal. This means that babies born from a father with scleroderma at no higher risk than other babies.

How scleroderma affects fertility in women

The good news is that the majority of women with scleroderma still experience normal fertility. However, women who develop scleroderma at a younger age are at a higher risk of infertility compared to older women who have already delivered children.

While a woman may experience normal fertility with scleroderma, there are higher risks associated with pregnancy particularly if a woman has a systemic form of scleroderma. The increased risk include:

- The development of pre-eclampsia, which is high blood pressure during pregnancy.

- Premature birth or babies born with low birth weight.

- Miscarriage.

- Kidney failure during pregnancy

- Difficulty placing drips or taking blood due to blood vessel involvement or skin thickening during labor and pregnancy.

- Difficulty acquiring general anesthesia if needed due to difficulties with mouth opening.

Any woman who is considering becoming pregnant after she has been diagnosed with scleroderma needs to ensure that preconception care is prioritized as part of her treatment plan. This firstly means a frank discussion with her physician who will refer her to a specialized rheumatologist and an obstetrician who is experienced in dealing with scleroderma and pregnancy. This will require an assessment of her current health to assess the risk of her and her baby if she were to become pregnant.

This is also important because it means that some drug treatments may need to be stopped or altered prior to the conception of a baby or within the early stages of pregnancy.

Most medical professionals advise that you do not contemplate pregnancy if you have serious lung, kidney or heart involvement. Also, women who have recently been diagnosed with scleroderma, which is within the last 4 years, are typically advised to delay pregnancy because pregnancy complications are typically higher in recent onset on scleroderma.

How to decrease the risk factors associated with pregnancy

After you have spoken to your doctor and have indeed decided to move forward with your pregnancy, here are a few tips to ensure that you have a safe a pregnancy, labor, and delivery as possible:

- Ensure that you are at a healthy weight to carry a baby to full term. Therefore, if you are overweight, speak to your doctor about developing a regiment for you to lose weight. If you are underweight, also discuss this with your doctor so that you can implement a plan to gain weight.

- Ensure that you eat a balanced diet and take dietary supplements if needed.

- Practice light exercise as long as it has been cleared by your doctor and do not overdo it.

- Take a daily dose of folic acid prior to conception and for the first 3 months of pregnancy.

- Speak to your doctor about taking a low dose of aspirin after 12 weeks of pregnancy to reduce the risk of developing pre-eclampsia.

- Do not use recreational drugs or alcohol, and do not smoke.

25

What is it like to be pregnant with scleroderma?

Typically, scleroderma patients have a straightforward pregnancy by virtue of the fact that most of them have normal pregnancies. This means that these women are typically not hospitalized during pregnancy. However, if complications do arise such as the development of preeclampsia or abnormalities in the baby's growth, the woman may need to be administered to the hospital for monitoring.

Pregnancy is a time filled with uncertainty, joy and excitement and most women, whether they suffer from scleroderma and not, have many questions. Below I will answer a few that are specific to women with scleroderma

How is a baby affected by scleroderma?

Most often babies are not affected by a mother's diagnosis with scleroderma. On the other hand, complications may arise if specific antibodies called anti-Ro, anti-La or antiphospholipid, cross from the scleroderma patient's bloodstream into the placenta and the baby's blood circulation. This can cause inflammation of the baby's heart in a condition known as heart block. If the mother has these antibodies in her bloodstream, a special test call a fetal echocardiogram is required during pregnancy to monitor the baby's heart as well as frequent monitoring.

Will scleroderma get worse during pregnancy?

While the majority of women do not experience further worsening of scleroderma during pregnancy, a few women have seen symptoms like increased skin thickening and itching. If you experience this, continue to use the solutions discussed earlier on to prevent and reduce this.

Also, women with a recent onset of kidney, lung, or heart involvement may see a worsening of these conditions. This is why it is vitally important that you be closely monitored by your doctor during pregnancy.

Another common symptom is heartburn but this is normal for all pregnancies. You can manage this symptom if you experience it during pregnancy by sitting upright while eating, eating slowly and using mild drugs that are safe during pregnancy such as ranitidine.

On the positive side, the symptoms of Raynaud's phenomenon may lessen or completely disappear during pregnancy because the condition increases internal body temperature and also increases blood flow to the toes and fingers.

Can a woman with scleroderma have a natural birth?

That is dependent on whether or not this woman had complications during her pregnancy and how severe her scleroderma symptoms are. The great news is that the majority of women are able to have natural births, especially if they delivered vaginally before being diagnosed with scleroderma. If scleroderma symptoms worsened during pregnancy or pregnancy complications such as preeclampsia developed, the doctor may advise that a woman deliver early with the use of drugs to induce labor or by caesarean section.

What happens after delivery?

Scleroderma patients may need to stay in the hospital a few days longer than other mothers if scleroderma symptoms flare-up or if there are complications during pregnancy, labor, or delivery.

Also, in a few cases, women find that their scleroderma symptoms worsen after having a baby. In such cases, doctors typically advise that they restart their pre-pregnancy medication immediately. Women with scleroderma should plan to have additional help after pregnancy because the trigger of scleroderma symptoms may require additional assistance while handling a baby.

Can scleroderma patients breastfeed?

Breastfeeding is the healthiest thing for any baby and is usually encouraged, even of scleroderma patients as most of the medication taken by scleroderma patients is safe to take during breastfeeding. This is something that needs to be discussed with your doctor especially if you suffer from Raynaud's phenomenon because Raynaud's symptoms can occur on the nipple. While this is typically not painful, it can be mistaken for other breastfeeding complications such as cracked nipples or thrush.

26

Should I consider HSCT (Hematopoietic Stem Cell Transplant)?

The cells of our body typically have specialized purposes and cannot be transformed into another type of cell with another purpose. For example, skin cells can only perform the function of skin cells and cannot, let's say, become cells that work efficiently in the eye.

Stem cells are different and have the potential to be developed into a wide variety of cells. This powerful characteristic allows stem cells to repair and maintain tissues and organs. They are also self-renewing and can produce more stem cells.

There are different types of stem cells. This differentiation is what allows different types of stem cells to perform specialized functions. The different types of stem cells are:

- Neural stem cells
- Epithelial stem cells
- Mesenchymal stem cells

- Hematopoietic stem cells

Due to the adaptive nature of stem cells, stem cell transplants have been under investigation for many years as a possible way to treat autoimmune diseases such as scleroderma. This investigation is based on the theory that stem cell transplant can modify or reset the immune system to reverse damage caused by scleroderma in tissues and organs.

The two stem cells of focus in these investigations are hematopoietic and mesenchymal stem cells. Hematopoietic stem cells have been the main focus in several clinical trials, particularly in patients with severe systemic scleroderma. Mesenchymal stem cells have not been studied as extensively even though early trials have suggested that they may have fewer side effects than hematopoietic stem cells but no large-scale clinical trials have been conducted so far.

Clinical tests conducted so far have been extremely encouraging. Particularly, the study titled, "Myeloablative Autologous Hematopoietic Stem Cell Transplantation for Severe Scleroderma: Long-Term Outcomes 6-11 Years after Entry on a Randomized Study Comparing Transplantation and Cyclophosphamide" was presented at the 2018 American College of Rheumatology (ACR)/Association of Reproductive Health Professionals (ARHP) and delivered results that stated that the majority of patients in the trial showed improved after transplant. The study showed that stem cell transplants work. Now, the search is on to find the answer of why.

- Therefore, while HSCT is a possibility for future scleroderma patients, it is not readily available for consideration by all scleroderma patients.

27

How do I deal with the mental trauma?

There is no evidence to support that scleroderma affects the central nervous system, however, there is no denying that patients who suffer from scleroderma often suffer from mood disorders, anxiety, depression, sexual dysfunction and altered self-image.

Scleroderma affects how we look and, therefore, affects the way that we feel about ourselves. Many scleroderma patients feel judged by other people because the symptoms of this disease sometimes cannot be hidden and dealt with in private.

Unfortunately, self-image is often a subject that is swept under the rug and is not addressed by a physician. Many scleroderma patients deal with this by socially isolating themselves but this only creates another problem as it affects this person's quality of life.

Therefore, it is imperative that scleroderma patients, and their support team including family members and medical doctor, realize that treating scleroderma does not only relate to the physical entities and outer appearance. A scleroderma patient's mental and emotional health also need to be managed. Ways in which this can be done include:

- Talking to someone. This can be another scleroderma patient who you can relate to or just someone who can provide a positive listening ear. Going to professional therapy sessions is also a great investment in your mental and emotional health.

- Writing down your emotions and the things that you are grateful for. Focusing on the things that you are grateful for improves your mental well-being and allows you to focus on the things that truly matter.

- Be mindful of the present moment so that you do not become overwhelmed by negative or difficult to deal with emotions. Pay attention to the physical sensations, tastes, smells and sounds around you so that you take joy in them rather than allow your mind to wander off to negativity.

- Exercise and partake in physical activities. The mood-boosting hormones that are released will certainly help make you feel better about your situation and yourself.

- Partake in activities that you love and explore new hobbies. Creative arts are a great form of expression and are also relaxing to perform.

- Make yourself laugh. Laughing reduces feelings of anxiety because it activates the release of feel-good hormones. You can make yourself laugh by watching a comedy movie, checking out funny videos on the internet or socializing with a funny friend or family member.

28

How much will I be affected by fatigue?

Fatigue is a common symptom of scleroderma and can be quite relentless as it is difficult to control and manage. Due to its obscure nature, it is something that is often overlooked compared to other possibly life-threatening symptoms such as lung involvement and heart failure.

Fatigue is no less important than other symptoms of scleroderma because it can be an indication of possible problems such as weakened immunity, lack of good sleep quality and quantity, being constantly in pain, and taking certain medications. Scleroderma patients who suffer from fatigue find that the most basic tasks require a huge amount of effort to perform. Activities such as getting dressed, walking up a flight of stairs, standing up for a few minutes, and bathing can require monumental strength and determination to do.

This can lead to chronic fatigue, which means that the sufferer hardly gets a reprieve from these feelings. Chronic fatigue displays symptoms such as:

- Being unable to get a good night's rest despite feeling tired.

- Feeling extremely exhausted night and day.

- Inability to concentrate and focus.

- Low productivity and efficiency.

- Disturbances in balance

- Pain and aches all over the body. Examples include joint pain, muscle soreness, and headaches.

Natural remedies for fighting the chronic fatigue of scleroderma

Of course, this is something that you need to discuss with your doctor so that a treatment option can be developed. However, there are a few natural remedies that may give you relief. They include:

- Valerian

- Licorice extract

- Ginseng

- Ginkgo

- Increasing vitamin B intake by eating foods such as bananas, sweet potatoes, hazelnut, cooked spinach, salmon, and tuna.

- Increasing magnesium and potassium intake by eating foods such as pumpkin seeds, spinach, dark chocolate, white beans, bananas, and mushrooms.

- Drinking herbal teas like ashwagandha, saw palmetto, green tea, chamomile, and lavender.

- Indulging in aromatherapy. Scents like peppermint oil are invigorating and helps boost energy.

Reducing caffeine and alcohol intake, reducing stress and exercise also help to combat fatigue. This last remedy is a little unconventional but some persons swear by its effectiveness. Lie on your back and prop your feet higher than your head with the help of pillows. This encourages blood flow to the brain, which boost alertness.

29

Are there any natural remedies that help with the symptoms of scleroderma?

There are a few common drugs such as glucocorticoids and penicillamine that are used to treat scleroderma but none of these drugs have a high degree of effectiveness. Many patients look to natural remedies to not only increase efficacy but to find relief from possible side effects of taking these drugs. This chapter discusses a few of the possible natural remedies that might work and how they work.

Potassium para-amino benzoic acid

Also known as PABA, this has anti-fibrosis qualities that are a result of its ability to increase oxygen absorption by tissues. This property has been acknowledged by the scientific community and, as such, this compound is found in several drugs that have a wide variety of therapeutic uses such as sunscreen, cancer therapy, and antibacterial. This compound can be obtained by indulging in a diet that includes grains, meat, and eggs

Vitamin E

Scleroderma patients experienced higher levels of oxidative stress compared to other people. Oxidative stress is an imbalance between antioxidants and free radicals.

Free radicals are molecules that are damaging to the cells of the body because of the highly reactive nature. This reactive nature causes a process called oxidation to occur. Oxidation strips healthy body cells and thus, causes damage. Antioxidants inhibit this process of oxidation. Vitamin E is a powerful antioxidant.

Foods that are rich in vitamin E include nuts like almonds and peanuts, seeds such as sunflower seeds, vegetables such as broccoli, kale and spinach, vegetable oils like soya bean and corn oil, and fortified breakfast cereals to name a few.

Vitamin E also helps keep the immune system strong so that it is protected against bacteria and viruses.

Vitamin C

Vitamin C is also known as ascorbic acid. It is also a powerful antioxidant that fights the oxidative process and discourages the presence of free radicals. Foods that are rich in vitamin C include fruits such as cantaloupe, orange, lemon, strawberry, and tomato, vegetables such as cauliflower and sweet potato, and herbs such as thyme and parsley.

Vitamin D

Patients who suffer from scleroderma are at a higher risk of developing osteoporosis. This risk can be reduced by increasing calcium intake. Calcium needs vitamin D to be absorbed and utilized efficiently by the body. Therefore, increasing vitamin D intake helps decrease the severity of bone-related scleroderma symptoms.

All you have to do to get vitamin D is step outside and soak up some sun. There are also vitamin D-rich foods such as dried mushrooms, tuna, mackerel, sardines, and salmon you can eat.

Evening primrose oil

This contains a high concentration of a compound called gamma-linolenic acid (GLA), which helps to reduce the symptoms of Raynaud's phenomenon. Evening primrose oil comes from its namesake which is a bi-annually weed found in North America and parts of Europe and Asia.

More natural remedies

Other natural remedies for scleroderma include estriol, n-acetylcysteine, bromelain, avocado oil, and soybean extract.

30

City or country living? Are some environments better suited for living with scleroderma?

As stated before one of the contributing factors to the development of scleroderma may be the environment that a person is exposed to. Chemical substances such as plastic certain drugs silicone organic solvents and silica powder common culprits. Silica exposure is frequent in areas where there are coal mining and sandblasting.

Other toxins in your environment that can trigger scleroderma symptoms include exposure to mercury, solvents such as those in paint thinners, cadmium and radiation.

As I speak of environment, I am not only speaking of external environment. Your internal environment matters just as much as your external environment. Artificial joints and silicone breast implants have also been shown to trigger scleroderma symptoms. You need to be mindful of what is in your body as much as what is out of it. Even some drugs and medications can induce scleroderma. Examples of these drugs include collagen and liquid silicone injections, cocaine and immunosuppressive drugs.

We all know that city and highly industrialized environments are notorious for have pollution that is filled with these kinds of chemicals and more.

If you are a person with scleroderma, you need to examine the environment that you live in and work in to determine whether it is a triggered your scleroderma diagnosis and symptoms. A few lifestyle changes that can be employed to detoxify your life of this triggering chemical and substances include:

- Changing living location if pollution and exposure to those mentioned above occur.

- Changing occupation if you work in a highly industrialized career and exposure to these chemicals and substances occurs.

- Removing silicone breast implants.

- Using safe solution products like paint thinners.

- Being mindful of fish and seafood sources to ensure that the fish and seafood you eat have low mercury content values.

Conclusion

Living healthy and happy with scleroderma is not easy but it is quite doable. This book was written to arm you with knowledge so that you do not become a victim of this disease but rather someone who triumphs over the symptoms.

The first step to combating this disease begins with diagnosis. With this diagnosis, you, your doctor and your support team can develop a comprehensive treatment plan that is personalized to you and your specific symptoms.

There are a lot of stigmas associated with any disease and the stigma can be quite intense with a condition like scleroderma where the symptoms such as discolored skin are so clearly visible for others to see and judge. Do not let that discourage you from finding the best treatment options for yourself.

Treating your scleroderma symptoms should include not only a physical regimen. This plan needs to include and encourage activities that boost mental and emotional health.

The key to being happy despite a scleroderma diagnosis is to realize that you are not defined by this disease. You are more than scleroderma. You are more than your symptoms. You are a person with a unique personality and so much to contribute to your community your family and the universe.

This book was written in an easy-to-follow we so that the confusion that often surrounds this illness is disbursed. It was written to give you clear and concise information and practical advice for managing scleroderma symptoms. I encourage you to reach out and let me know how the words within this book have helped you. We scleroderma patients need to stick together and support each other because we alone know the difficulties we face.

Thank you for purchasing this book. I hope that you see great improvement in your health and your management of this disease. Also, if you enjoyed this content, then kindly leave a review on Amazon.com. Your feedback does mean a lot to me!

References

Anbiaee, N., & Tafakhori, Z. (2011). Early diagnosis of progressive systemic sclerosis (scleroderma) from a panoramic view: report of three cases. *Dento maxillo facial radiology, 40*(7), 457–462. https://doi.org/10.1259/dmfr/64340754

Marek, M., & Rudny, R. (2016). Scleroderma of geriatric age and scleroderma-like paraneoplastic syndrome - description of two cases. *Reumatologia, 54*(2), 91–94. https://doi.org/10.5114/reum.2016.60220

Pattanaik, D., Brown, M., Postlethwaite, B. C., & Postlethwaite, A. E. (2015). Pathogenesis of Systemic Sclerosis. *Frontiers in immunology, 6*, 272. https://doi.org/10.3389/fimmu.2015.00272

Shah, A. A., & Wigley, F. M. (2013). My approach to the treatment of scleroderma. *Mayo Clinic proceedings, 88*(4), 377–393. https://doi.org/10.1016/j.mayocp.2013.01.018

Sobolewski, P., Maślińska, M., Wieczorek, M., Łagun, Z., Malewska, A., Roszkiewicz, M., Nitskovich, R., Szymańska, E., & Walecka, I. (2019). Systemic sclerosis - multidisciplinary disease: clinical features and treatment. *Reumatologia, 57*(4), 221–233. https://doi.org/10.5114/reum.2019.87619

Young, A., & Khanna, D. (2015). Systemic sclerosis: commonly asked questions by rheumatologists. *Journal of clinical rheumatology : practical reports on rheumatic & musculoskeletal diseases, 21*(3), 149–155. https://doi.org/10.1097/RHU.0000000000000232

Made in the USA
Middletown, DE
02 October 2020